P9-CMX-245

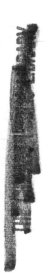

	DATE DUE	

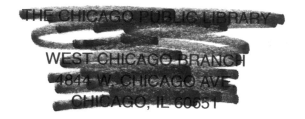

Everything You Need to Know About

The Dangers of Cosmetic Surgery

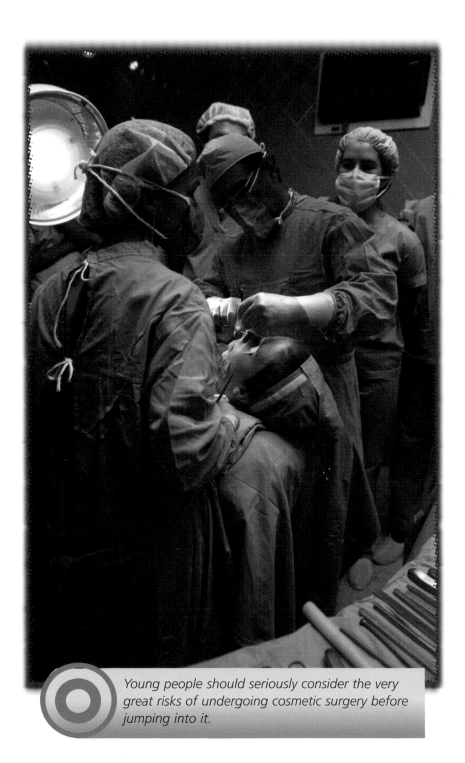

Young people should seriously consider the very great risks of undergoing cosmetic surgery before jumping into it.

Everything You Need to Know About The Dangers of Cosmetic Surgery

Magdalena Alagna

The Rosen Publishing Group, Inc.
New York

Published in 2002 by The Rosen Publishing Group, Inc.
29 East 21st Street, New York, NY, 10010

The people pictured in this book are only models. They in no way practice or endorse the activities illustrated. Captions serve only to explain the subjects of photographs and do not in any way imply a connection between the real-life models and the staged situations.

Library of Congress Cataloging-in-Publication Data

Alagna, Magdalena.
Everything you need to know about the dangers of cosmetic surgery / by Magdalena Alagna.
p. cm. — (The need to know library)
Includes bibliographical references and index.
ISBN 0-8239-3552-3
1. Surgery, Plastic—Complications—Juvenile literature.
[1. Surgery, Plastic.] I. Title. II. Series.
RD118.7 .A42 2002
617.9'5—dc21

2002002067

Manufactured in the United States of America

Contents

Introduction

Teens are the most controversial new category of plastic surgery patients. Although teens are not in the majority of those who get cosmetic surgery, more teens are getting cosmetic surgery than ever before. In 1999, 1,645 patients eighteen and younger had liposuction, and 1,840 had their breasts enlarged. That's twice as many as in 1992!

Why are so many teens getting cosmetic surgery? Plastic surgeon Dr. Edward Domanskis, of Newport Beach, California, said of teen cosmetic surgery in a 1998 article in the *American Medical News*: "Although teen cosmetic surgery is very controversial, the pressures of looking good have resulted in a steady increase in that age group seeking procedures such as nose reshaping, breast reduction, and liposuction."

More than half of the people who get plastic surgery are under thirty-five. The number of teens who get cosmetic surgery is growing. With the growth of such a trend comes an increase in the concerns adults have about teen cosmetic surgery. Researcher Kearney Cooke said, "What's most disturbing to me is that this is a time when their bodies aren't fully formed, yet teens feel so much pressure to be instantly perfect."

Figures from the American Society of Plastic Surgeons (ASPS) show a big increase in the number of cosmetic surgery patients in the United States. The number of cosmetic surgery procedures reported by board-certified plastic surgeons grew from 367,000 in 1992 to 900,000 in 1998 and to 1.1 million in 1999. These numbers may represent only part of the total. Many ASPS-recognized doctors are too busy to report to the organization.

Popular Procedures

Nationwide, the most popular procedure is liposuction (lipoplasty), regardless of how dangerous it is. "To put it in perspective, the incidence of death from liposuction is two to three times higher than that of dying from a normal pregnancy," said Robert del Junco, former president of the California State Medical Board in an October 2000 article in *People* magazine.

Other popular procedures include breast augmentation, eyelid surgery (blepharoplasty), tummy tucks (abdominoplasty), and face-lifts (rhytidectomy). Also high on the list are hair transplants, laser hair removal, skin resurfacing, dermabrasion skin work, pinning back ears (otoplasty), and penile enlargement (phalloplasty).

More men are having cosmetic surgery than ever, according to a study done by the American Society of Plastic and Reconstructive Surgeons. The 1998 study shows that in the five years prior to the study, male face-lifts had doubled. In 1999, the ASPS reported that almost 11 percent of all cosmetic surgery procedures were performed on men. Men are going in droves to sur-geons for eyelid surgery, face-lifts, and liposuction to get rid of their "spare tires." Nose reshaping (rhinoplasty), breast reduction, liposuction, eyelid surgery, and face-lifts are among the top five cosmetic surgery procedures for men, according to the ASPS.

Consider the Risks

Who are the doctors doing cosmetic surgery? Are there agencies to regulate the standard of care for such proce-dures? Doctors, and even spas, that perform many cos-metic procedures advertise cosmetic surgery as though it is no more difficult, painful, time consuming, or expen-sive than getting a facial. However, cosmetic surgery has the emphasis on surgery. The results can be fatal.

The risks go beyond the more immediate physical dan-ger. Cosmetic surgery is expensive. Because it is elective surgery, many health insurance companies do not cover the costs. That means consumers must pay out of their own pockets. Cosmetic surgery can run into the thousands of dollars, and many people finance the surgeries no matter what the cost. These people are led on by the goal of perfection as it is pitched to them by movies, television, magazines, billboards, and the advertising that brings home the message that our culture does not value anyone but the thin, the young, and the attractive.

What is the role of advertising in cosmetic surgery? "There's a considerable amount of deception and outright fraud by doctors whose greed far exceeds their scruples and surgical skills," said Dr. Mark Gorney, former president of the ASPS. "Patients pay with their looks, sometimes even their lives, because a slick ad lures them into the wrong hands." Cosmetic surgery is even being auctioned off on the Internet!

In fact, the state of California is so worried about sleazy advertising campaigns that it passed a law in January 2000 banning inflated credentials, false scientific claims, deceptive before-and-after pictures, misleading testimonials, and statements that downplay the risks and pain of procedures. As part of this law, doctors may not claim they are "board certified" unless they specify which board certified them.

Advertisements not only entice people to get one procedure done, but they also convey the general tone

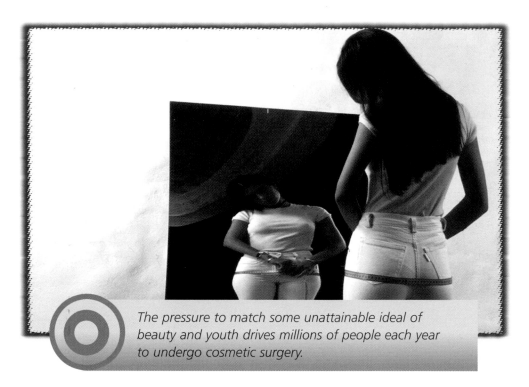

The pressure to match some unattainable ideal of beauty and youth drives millions of people each year to undergo cosmetic surgery.

that more plastic surgery is better. This is especially dangerous because the more procedures that are done, the longer you are on the operating table, and the greater the risk.

What are the most common cosmetic surgeries? What are the risks associated with them? In this book you will find out that the dangers of cosmetic surgery far outweigh any possible benefits. You should always keep in mind whether you are willing to die for an image of perfection pushed on you by standards created in an advertising boardroom or a fashion magazine photo shoot. Remember, too, that disfigurement is an all-too-common result of cosmetic surgery. There are many, many stories of cosmetic surgery disasters.

What You Should Know

First you should be aware that not all of the people performing cosmetic surgery procedures are experienced in doing them. Some aren't even trained to do them. Second, you should know that the risks happen far more often than anyone realizes. This is because many of the procedures are done in doctors' offices and the statistics are not reported. Third, you should not believe that the newer, "safer" cosmetic surgery techniques mean that cosmetic surgery is safe. Every advance in cosmetic surgery brings with it a significant risk specific to the procedures. Also, the risks of surgery are always present, no matter how evolved the new techniques are.

There are countless stories of people who have become disfigured or whose health has declined as a result of cosmetic surgery. These stories sound like science fiction, but they are terribly real: A woman unable to close her eyes or smile anymore as a result of a botched face-lift. A man with a gaping hole in the shaft of his penis as a result of a penile enlargement. A woman with dead, black skin peeling off her legs as a result of skin tissue death from a liposuction procedure.

What is cosmetic surgery, exactly? How is it commonly used? What are the dangers of cosmetic surgery? This book will answer all of these questions, and more.

Chapter 1

Why Cosmetic Surgery?

Why do people get cosmetic surgery? A quick look at some of the most popular procedures will illustrate that the main reason people get cosmetic surgery is because they are dissatisfied with their appearances. People get liposuction on every area of the face and body that you can name. Liposuction is the removal of fat. People get fat sucked from under their eyes to make the bags under their eyes go away. They get the fat sucked from under their cheekbones to make their cheekbones more defined. They get fat sucked from their abdomens to get rid of a spare tire or love handles.

Also, many young people get breast augmentation, or breast implants. You may have heard about the grave danger of getting silicone-filled breast implants. You may think that the new, saline-filled implants are a safer alternative. Don't be fooled. Cosmetic surgery is a dangerous risk to take. Any surgery comes with a set of risk factors.

Body Image Standards

In a recent study done by *Seventeen* magazine, nearly half of the fourteen- to eighteen-year-olds surveyed said they were dissatisfied with their bodies, and a third of the teens said they were considering some type of plastic surgery. People want to improve their appearances because they may believe their flaws are worse than they actually are. In its most severe form, this is called body dysmorphic disorder. But our perception of our appearance may have nothing to do with the way others see us. Instead it may have more to do with the advertising with which we are surrounded every day. Consider the advertisements on television, in magazines, and on billboards, to name a few places, that use beautiful people to sell products. These advertisements increase the chance that someone who looks fine, who is in fact perfectly fit, could feel dissatisfied with his or her body.

Remember, too, that the cosmetic industry, the business of beauty, is a big business. Many companies have lots of money invested in fueling unrealistic expectations of how people should look. Therefore, the message is everywhere. Turn on the television, and there are numerous advertisements for gyms and weight-loss programs.

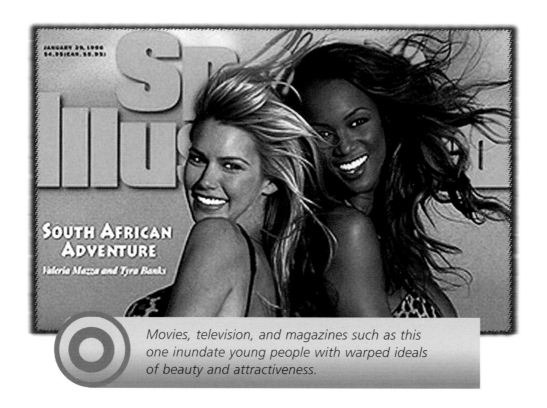

JANUARY 29, 1996
$4.95(CAN. $5.95)

SOUTH AFRICAN
ADVENTURE

Valeria Mazza and Tyra Banks

Movies, television, and magazines such as this one inundate young people with warped ideals of beauty and attractiveness.

Turn on the radio and the same commercials are there. It is hard to escape the media blitz telling you that you should look different than how you do.

The Pressure to Be Attractive and Thin

Why do people get cosmetic surgery? One big reason is that they want to be attractive, whatever that means to them. They want luscious lips like their favorite movie star's, so they get collagen injected into their lips. They want a flatter stomach, so they get a tummy tuck. Another reason is that people want to be thin. This is an especially dangerous part of body image because the desire to be thin has caused near-epidemic proportions of eating disorders, as well as terrible cosmetic surgery disasters.

Some people get cosmetic surgery because they want to express themselves, and they do so by altering their appearances. Body modification has gotten much attention in recent years. Some of the procedures, such as putting metal plates in the head or the face, for instance, or getting small horns implanted in the skin of the scalp, definitely count as cosmetic surgery.

It is important to remember, in this looks-conscious society, that real health may have little to do with what we see as the appearance of health or beauty. If you have ever considered plastic surgery, ask yourself what the main reason is. Chances are that you may feel the need to reach some standard of beauty that is totally unrealistic and that has little to do with health.

What Is Real Health?

In 1985, the World Health Organization (WHO) defined health as involving complete physical, social, and psychological well-being and not just the absence of disease. This means that we must look at the quality-of-life standards for individuals when examining the desire for cosmetic surgery.

Many people who want to get plastic surgery are convinced that they cannot have either the social life they want or the psychological health and confidence they desire, unless they have plastic surgery. There is some question as to whether the screening processes most doctors have for patients are adequate to identify patients' psychological health as it influences their desire to have cosmetic surgery.

To be in line with the WHO's standards of health, it is important for each of us to strive for positive self-image, which will assist us in forming a social support network of friends and family members who wish us well and have our best interests at heart. It isn't always easy to achieve a positive self-image in this culture that bombards us with unrealistic images of beauty. However, there are plenty of people who manage to feel good about themselves, without placing their lives in jeopardy by undergoing cosmetic surgery!

The Food and Drug Administration (FDA) has published its health guidelines in the form of the food guide pyramid. The pyramid shows the four food groups and how many servings one should eat from each group per day. The food guide pyramid also explains what makes a serving. In addition to following the food guide pyramid, it is well-known that everyone should exercise at least for a little while every day. If you eat a moderate, well-balanced diet and get enough exercise, that will be all you need to do to stay and look healthy.

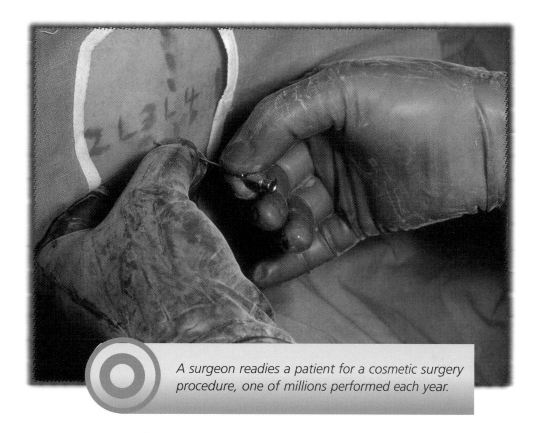

A surgeon readies a patient for a cosmetic surgery procedure, one of millions performed each year.

Statistics on Cosmetic Surgery

In the 1998 study by the American Society of Plastic and Reconstructive Surgeons, statistics showed that the number of liposuctions has tripled; the numbers of most other cosmetic procedures have increased as well. The number of breast implants has more than doubled since 1992.

Even plastic surgeons agree that such statistics may not tell the whole story of adolescent cosmetic surgery. This is because many more procedures are being done in a doctor's office instead of a hospital. It is likely that many of these surgeries done in doctors' offices are not reported.

Teen Cosmetic Surgery

Dr. Edward Domanskis, a surgeon who has a personal Web site where he conducts online consultations with patients, said that he receives a lot of e-mail from teenagers inquiring about cosmetic surgery. He said, "In our society, there is no such thing as being too thin. A pre-occupation with the body and a constant focus on small flaws can become an obsession with teens."

Nor is it just the teenagers themselves who may have the idea to get plastic surgery. Dr. Domanskis recalled the case of a nineteen-year-old woman who came to a cosmetic surgeon for breast augmentation. After consultation, it was clear that it was the woman's mother who wanted her daughter to get the surgery so that the daughter's breasts would match her sister's. The doctor performed the surgery, but the mother was still unsatisfied, and so the girl went through another procedure. Many doctors must question, when faced with a prospective client who is a teenager, who it is who really wants the surgery—the child or the parents.

It Could Happen to You

South Florida's *Sun-Sentinel* did an extensive survey of cosmetic surgery. It tracked deaths and complications from plastic surgery using computerized Florida Department of Insurance medical malpractice claims data, lawsuits, autopsy findings, media reports, and

Cosmetic Surgery Disaster

Jeanette Mordica, forty-four years old, went into the doctor's office for liposuction and a tummy tuck on March 28, 1997. She was dead the next day. Jeanette Mordica was five feet tall and weighed 162 pounds, and she had hoped that cosmetic surgery would do for her what failed dieting and exercise had never done.

Her surgery lasted for five hours and was performed without complications. She stayed in the hospital overnight and woke up the next day with no problems. During the course of the day, she told the nurses that she felt dizziness and a shortness of breath, and that her heart was racing. She went into cardiac arrest. The *Sun-Sentinel*, a regional newspaper covering southern Florida, quoted Dr. Richard Edison, one of the doctors who worked at the facility where Jeanette Mordica got her surgery: "Unfortunately, these are problems that occur with a small percentage of cases." Doctors at the facility agreed that there was no way her death could have been prevented.

The medical examiner ruled that her death was from pulmonary thromboemboli, or blood clots that form in the lungs. Thromboembolism is a complication of both liposuction and tummy-tuck surgery.

Florida Board of Medicine disciplinary-action records. The research showed that death occurred in both men and women of all ages and from all economic classes. The causes were varied. They could be anything from complications in breast implant surgery for young women to face-lifts for elderly men.

Autopsy reports didn't really explain whether any of these deaths could have been prevented. In some cases, it was clear that the deceased had been victims of poor surgical techniques. However, some autopsy reports suggested that the doctors did not properly evaluate the patients' general health before the surgery. Certain factors, such as age, weight, heart problems, or cigarette smoking, are risk factors in any surgery.

The *Sun-Sentinel* also analyzed 1,100 plastic surgery malpractice claims filed with the state insurance department. The injured victims spanned all age groups, though a little more than half were women in their late thirties. Injuries could be anything from temporary loss of feeling in a body part to serious, permanent damage. For example, a forty-six-year-old woman had surgery to improve the size and lift of her breasts. She lost both nipples after the breast tissue died. She had to get three more operations and a breast reconstruction.

In the next chapter, we will take a look at exactly what cosmetic surgery is and how it differs from other methods used to improve the appearance, and we will take a good look at some of the most common procedures.

Chapter 2

What Is Cosmetic Surgery?

Most plastic surgery developments happened during World War I. World War I was the first time that surgeons saw so many terrible facial and head injuries, caused by weapons such as poison gas, machine guns, and grenades. This challenged surgeons to develop new skills and procedures. By the 1950s and 1960s, doctors had learned to do breast jobs and tummy tucks. Liposuction was developed in the 1970s.

How Cosmetic Surgery Differs from Plastic and Reconstructive Surgery

According to the ASPS, there are differences among plastic surgery, reconstructive surgery, and cosmetic surgery. Plastic surgery is surgery dealing with the repair of injured, deformed, or destroyed parts of the body. Often this involves transferring skin and bone from other parts of the body or from another person. For example, some-one who was in a car accident may have had extensive injury to his face. A plastic surgeon might take pieces of bone from another part of the person's body to recon-struct the damaged cheekbone and jaw.

Reconstructive surgery is a type of plastic surgery. It is performed on abnormal structures caused by congeni-tal defects (defects that you were born with), develop-mental defects, trauma (when you've been in an accident), infection, tumors, or disease.

Cosmetic surgery is surgery that is performed to reshape normal structures of the body. For instance, there may not be anything medically wrong with your nose, but you want to get cosmetic surgery so that your nose looks more attractive to you.

Some Common Cosmetic Surgery Procedures

Abdominoplasty

Abdominoplasty, more commonly called a tummy tuck, is a surgical procedure during which excess skin and fat are removed from the abdomen. Muscles also may be tightened. A horizontal cut is made in the abdomen at the level of the pubic hair. The abdominal muscles

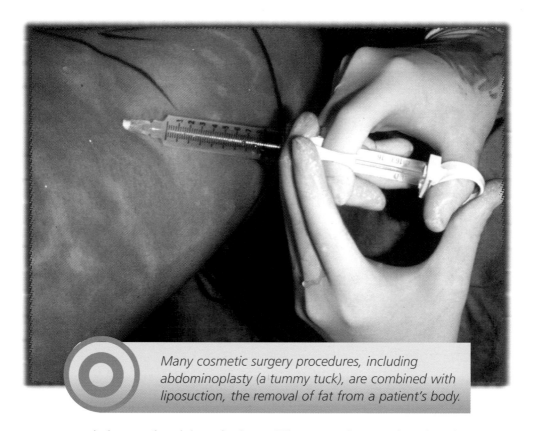

Many cosmetic surgery procedures, including abdominoplasty (a tummy tuck), are combined with liposuction, the removal of fat from a patient's body.

are tightened with stitches. The navel remains in the same place but must be brought out through another opening in the skin. That means that the navel gets covered over with skin when the skin shifts during the operation. To make the navel visible again, the doctor has to cut a hole in the skin covering the navel and pull it from under the skin to the top layer of the skin, where it can be seen again. Liposuction of the hips often is performed with abdominoplasty.

Blepharoplasty

Blepharoplasty, or eyelid surgery, is a common cosmetic procedure performed on many teenagers. This procedure extends the eyelid, giving the patient a more wide-eyed appearance. Many people think that this wide-eyed look makes a person appear younger, fresher, and smarter. This procedure is performed by making cuts in the natural contour lines of the upper eyelid.

Breast Augmentation

Breast augmentation surgery is one of the most popular surgeries for teens. A 1999 article in *Newsweek* magazine quoted Amber Reeves, a high-school junior, as saying, "A lot of seniors at my school get breast augmentation as a graduation present."

At first, breast implants were used mostly for breast cancer patients who had had mastectomies. Many of the early breast implants, those done in the 1960s, used an implant that was a rubber silicone envelope filled with silicone gel. Only about 10 percent were filled with saline (salt water). Today, most breast implants are saline-filled implants.

Dermabrasion

Dermabrasion is the process of scraping away the outer layers of skin. The surgeon scrapes until the level of skin is reached that will make a scar less visible. This is done to allow new skin to grow. Surgeons use a rough wire brush that is attached to a motorized handle. This procedure is often done to correct acne scars or other scarring.

Liposuction

Liposuction is a procedure that sucks the fat out of a part of the body. How is this done? Usually, the doctor begins the surgery by drawing lines on the patient's skin. Then the patient is put under general anesthesia. Sometimes the doctor runs an ultrasound wand over the site of the liposuction to liquefy the fat. That makes the fat easier to remove. Then the doctor inserts a tube about the size of a ballpoint pen into the site and vacuums the fat into a beaker.

With tumescent liposuction, the doctor floods the fat with fluids. This makes the suction easier and lets the doctor take out more fat. Tumescent liposuction is also called "wet" liposuction. The fluid contains epinephrine (adrenaline), which constricts blood vessels and reduces bleeding. It also contains lidocaine, an anesthetic, which gives enough pain control that a patient may not need general anesthesia.

Otoplasty

Otoplasty, or ear pinning, is a popular surgery for children and for teens. Otoplasty is done by making cuts behind the ears that lay open the cartilage of the ear. Then the doctor can stitch the cartilage together or can remove excess cartilage. Lastly the doctor stitches the skin of the ears into place. This kind of surgery can be performed on anyone six years or older. It may require a stay in the hospital, or it may be done in a doctor's office.

The risks of the procedure are the same risks that go for any surgery, which will be discussed in the next chapter.

Phalloplasty

Phalloplasty, or penis enlargement, is done to accomplish two goals. The first is to make the penis appear longer. Penile lengthening procedures usually make the penis appear noticeably longer only in its flaccid (soft) state. The second goal is to make the penis wider.

There are some experimental techniques used to increase the girth, or width, of the penis. Some of these techniques include injecting fat from other parts of the body into the penis, or carving strips of fat from a person's buttocks or thighs and then injecting them into cuts made in the shaft of the penis. Some men try to increase the girth of the penis by getting collagen injections, even though collagen can cause allergic reactions.

How is penile lengthening done? The surgeon makes an incision in the abdomen above where the penis attaches to the body. The ligament is snipped that supports penile erection. The "inner penis" is then tugged away from the bone. Once the wound heals, the penis hangs lower.

Plumping

Plumping is the common name for collagen injections into certain parts of the body, often the lips, to make them appear fuller. Collagen is inserted with an injection beneath the skin of the part of the body that is being "plumped." Collagen is a liquid made from the connective tissue of cows or pigs. Injectable collagen is used for filling in "contour deformities" in the skin, such as acne scars or wrinkles. But the FDA has not approved it for enlarging facial features, such as lips.

Reduction Mammaplasty

Both women and men get reduction mammaplasty, or breast reductions. When men have large breasts, the condition is called gynecomastia. The word "gynecomastia" comes from a Greek word meaning "womenlike breasts." According to the ASPS, it's actually quite a common condition, affecting an estimated 40 to 60 percent of men, many of whom choose to have breast reduction.

Breast reductions are performed when a person's breasts are unusually large for his or her body size. The breast reduction procedure removes fat and glandular tissue, and in some cases excess skin, from the breasts, leaving them smaller and more firm.

Rhinoplasty

Rhinoplasty is the name cosmetic surgeons give to nose reshaping. This is the most common aesthetic procedure requested by teens, according to the American Society for Aesthetic Plastic Surgery. It can be performed when the nose has completed 90 percent of its growth, which can occur as young as age thirteen or fourteen in girls and fifteen or sixteen in boys. Procedures in rhinoplasty vary. Surgeons can shave off a bone to get rid of a bump, place nasal implants to lengthen the nose, cut wide nostrils, raise the tip of the nose, get rid of a hooked nose, and reshape the nose bridge.

How is it done? First, the doctor separates the skin of the nose from the underlying bone and cartilage. The bone and cartilage are then reshaped, and the skin is redraped over the surface. Sometimes the bone is broken, but that is not as common as it used to be.

Rhytidectomy

The medical term for a face-lift is rhytidectomy. What is a face-lift? It is a surgical procedure that removes excess fat, tightens underlying facial muscles, and redrapes the skin of the face. It does not improve the appearance of sagging eyelids or foreheads, or baggy neck skin, so many people get surgery on those areas as well as getting a face-lift.

A face-lift is done by making cuts above the hairline at the temples, extending the cut in front of the ear or inside the cartilage at the front of the ear, and then continuing behind the earlobe to the lower scalp. Then the surgeon separates the skin from the fat and muscle below. Fat can be trimmed or sucked from around the neck and chin. The surgeon then tightens the underlying muscle and pulls the skin back, removing the extra skin. This gives the skin of the face a tighter appearance.

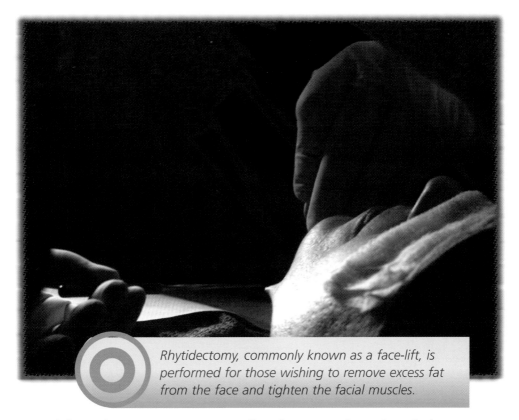

Rhytidectomy, commonly known as a face-lift, is performed for those wishing to remove excess fat from the face and tighten the facial muscles.

After the surgery, a small tube may be placed (temporarily) under the skin behind the ear to drain any blood that might collect there. The surgeon also may wrap the head with bandages to try to minimize the bruising and swelling.

Do you still think that cosmetic surgery is a simple cosmetic procedure and not a surgical procedure filled with risk factors? Read on to find out more about the risks of any surgery and about the special risks associated with cosmetic surgery.

Chapter 3

The Risks of Cosmetic Surgery

Now that you know a little bit more about how some of the most common procedures are done, cosmetic surgery may not seem like such a great option anymore. Cosmetic surgery procedures claim to enhance attractiveness in an almost magical fashion. The truth of the matter is that cosmetic surgery is a surgical procedure like any other.

General Surgical Risks

All surgeries have some degree of risk. These include bleeding, infection, anesthesia reaction, or unexpected scarring. There could also be hematoma (collection of blood at the surgical site) or seroma (collection of fluid at the surgical site).

Other possible complications of surgery include nausea, vomiting, and fever, as well as hemorrhaging (heavy or uncontrolled bleeding), thrombosis (abnormal clotting), and skin necrosis, which is skin tissue death as a result of not enough blood flow to the skin.

Risks Associated with Cosmetic Surgery

There are risks to any surgery, but there are some specific risks associated with cosmetic surgery. These risk factors are a result of the surgical techniques used, the process of the surgery, and the areas of the body on which the work is being done.

In the *Gale Encyclopedia of Medicine*, the risks of cosmetic surgery are described as:

◎ **Wound infection**

◎ **Internal bleeding**

◎ **Pneumonia**

◎ **Reactions to the anesthesia**

◎ **Formation of undesirable scar tissue**

◎ **Persistent pain, redness, or swelling in the area of surgery**

◎ **Anemia (lowering of the red blood cell count, which makes a person very weak)**

◎ **Fat embolisms (when fat cells travel through the body and lodge somewhere) from liposuction**

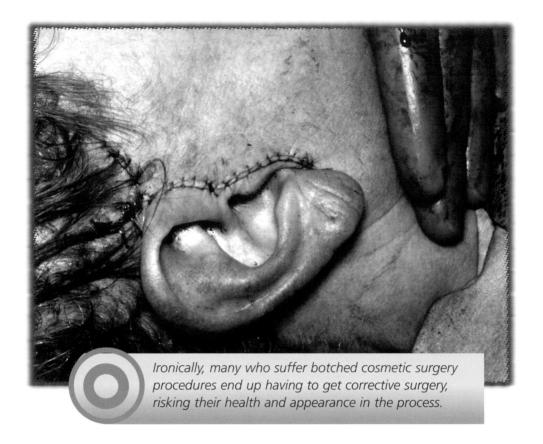

Ironically, many who suffer botched cosmetic surgery procedures end up having to get corrective surgery, risking their health and appearance in the process.

- ◎ Rejection of skin grafts or tissue transplants

- ◎ Loss of normal feeling or function in the area of operation

- ◎ Complications resulting from unforeseen technological problems

In addition, some of the other complications of cosmetic surgery are:

◎ Crusting along the incision lines.

◎ Numbness. Small sensory nerves under the skin are occasionally cut when the incision is made or interrupted by undermining of the skin during surgery. Sometimes the sensitivity never returns.

◎ Scars. All new scars are red, dark pink, or purple. Scars on the body may take a year or longer to fade completely. Sometimes you may have to get more cosmetic surgery to get rid of ugly scars.

◎ Abnormal scars. Injection of steroids into the scars, placement of silicone sheeting onto the scars, or further surgery to correct the scars may be necessary.

◎ Injury to deeper structures such as blood vessels, nerves, and muscles.

Medical complications such as pulmonary embolism (blockage of an artery in the lung), severe allergic reactions to medications, cardiac arrhythmia (when your heart beats irregularly), heart attack, and hyperthermia (uncontrollable fever) are some of the serious and life-threatening risks of cosmetic surgery.

No one knows how often cosmetic surgery proves fatal, since risk data are not compiled in a central clearinghouse.

Outpatient Cosmetic Surgery Is Actually the Riskier Choice

Many patients find that the promise of outpatient surgery is more comforting than a hospital stay. However, it is the outpatient surgery that can be riskiest. Remember that hospitals are required to meet strict equipment and personnel guidelines. That just may not be the case with a doctor's office. There have been numerous stories of cosmetic surgery patients who died because the doctors' offices did not have the equipment that was needed to save their lives, and that a hospital definitely would have had on hand immediately.

If cosmetic surgery is being performed in a doctor's office, there might not be an anesthesiologist there, although anesthesia should be given only by a trained anesthesiologist. Even if there is an anesthesiologist present, receiving anesthesia is still a tricky business. What are some of the things that can happen during surgery because of wrongly administered anesthesia? Results can include brain damage, nerve damage, eye damage, stroke, burn, myocardial infarction (irreversible injury to the heart muscle), and death.

Risks Associated with Some of the Most Common Procedures

Abdominoplasty

With this type of surgery, you run the risk of blood clots, infection, bleeding under the skin, and poor healing resulting in noticeable scarring or skin loss. Blood clots are what happen when blood coagulates, or thickens. Blood clots can lodge in a part of the body and block off the supply of blood or oxygen to the part, resulting in a host of problems. In addition, you can contract necrotising fasicitis, a potentially fatal infection. There also is the risk of peritonitus, which is what happens when the abdominal muscle gets punctured.

Blepharoplasty

The risks of this type of surgery include hemorrhaging, infection, unfavorable external scar, blindness, ectropion (retraction of the lower lid), persistent dry eyes, irritation in the cornea, not enough skin left (meaning you must get a skin graft), asymmetry, sensitivity to light, numbness, itching, and reaction to medications.

Breast Augmentation

Any breast augmentation poses the risk of asymmetry, meaning that the breasts could be two different sizes and you will have to undergo surgery again to make the breasts look symmetrical. Persistent pain is another potential complication.

A thick scar, also called a capsule, can form around the implant, as part of the body's normal reaction to a foreign substance. When the scar becomes firm, or hardens, that is called capsular contracture. This may cause pain. It also may change the texture and appearance of the breast.

Implants also can rupture and leak. They can deflate, or they can become displaced. The chances of capsular contracture or rupture increase with the age of the implant. If one of these complications occurs, you will have to have outpatient surgery to loosen the capsule or remove or replace the implant.

Other risks include joint pain and swelling, skin tightness, swelling of hands and feet, rash, swollen glands or lymph nodes, unusual fatigue, general aching, viruses and flu, unusual hair loss, memory problems, headaches, muscle weakness or burning, nausea or vomiting, irritable bowel syndrome, and a greater chance of getting colds. In addition, all implants must be removed or replaced after a number of years.

When you get a mammogram, which is used to test women for breast cancer or any other illness or abnormality in the breast tissue, you have to get a special kind of mammogram to move implants away from the breast tissue. It is important to remember that this could interfere with detecting breast cancer by "hiding" a suspicious lesion (spot). Also, it may be hard for the doctor reading

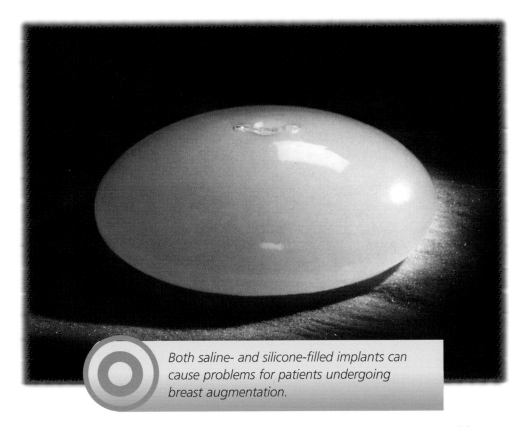

Both saline- and silicone-filled implants can cause problems for patients undergoing breast augmentation.

the mammogram to tell whether you have a tumor or if you just have calcium deposits formed in the scar tissue from the breast implant.

There can be either temporary or permanent change or loss of sensation in the nipple or breast tissue. Silicone has been linked to increased symptoms for connective tissue diseases such as arthritis.

Dermabrasion

The patient must avoid direct sunlight for six to twelve months while the skin's pigmentation (coloring) returns. There is the danger of permanent skin color changes, infection, scarring, flare-up of skin allergies, fever blisters, and cold sores. The smoothing effects of the surgery are said to be permanent, but they do not prevent new skin eruptions from being formed. In some cases, heart irregularities could occur.

Liposuction

A recent controversial study published in the medical journal *Plastic and Reconstructive Surgery* reported that, based on a survey of doctors, the death rate for liposuction was an alarming 1 in 5,000. This compares to a death rate of about 1 in 30,000 for a hernia operation.

Patients often donate their own blood prior to surgery in case a transfusion is required. You could have difficulty breathing during or even after the surgery. The cause could be anything from allergic reaction to heart failure. In addition, sometimes pieces of fat can break off and go floating through the bloodstream. This is called a fat embolus, and it poses many of the same health risks that blood clots do.

You run the risk of infection, clots, fluid accumulation, skin loss, perforation of organs, pain, swelling, bleeding, numbness, rippled or baggy skin, uneven pigmentation, asymmetry, and scarring. Liposuction can cause fluid buildup in the lungs and fatal blood clots. Also, patients can lose too much fluid during the suctioning process, sending them into shock.

Some fluid that is pumped into the body during wet liposuction is suctioned back out with the fat, but most is absorbed into your blood. This can result in congestive heart failure and pulmonary edema (fluid in the lungs), both potentially fatal. Finally, one of the risks of wet liposuction is that too much epinephrine can be flooded into your system, which could lead to cardiac arrest.

Phalloplasty

The loss of support from when the ligament is cut can lower the angle of the erection. The newly exposed shaft portion of the penis may be covered by unwanted pubic hair. The ligament can reattach to the pubic bone and retract (pull back) the penis farther inside than it was before. Other complications may include infection, scarring, cosmetic deformity, sexual dysfunction, and shrinkage. "Penile augmentation procedures are unsafe, primarily because the outcome is unpredictable and any patient can end up with a shorter penis instead of a longer penis," said Dr. Jack McAninch, president of the American Urological Association.

The American Urological Association has declared fat injection and cutting the suspensory ligament in the penis neither safe nor effective. The American Society for Aesthetic Plastic Surgery says that penile fat injection is experimental, with "insufficient data to establish its safety and effectiveness."

"The deformities are significant. The scarring that results is significant," said Dr. McAninch.

Plumping

The use of collagen injections has been associated with connective tissue diseases. The FDA is still investigating how often people get connective tissue diseases after getting collagen injections.

The risks are that you may be allergic to collagen and not even know it. This could take the form of a rash, hives, joint and muscle pain, headache, and severe reactions that include shock and difficulty breathing. Other bad effects that have occurred after collagen injections include infections, abscesses, open sores, lumps, peeling of the skin, scarring, recurrence of herpes simplex, and partial blindness.

Reduction Mammaplasty

Breast reduction surgery, although beneficial for some people, also carries many risks. As with breast augmentation, there is a chance that the breasts will be asymmetrical. Swelling, pain, bruising, and scarring are definite results of the surgery. Hematomas (collection of blood under the skin), seromas (collection of fluid under the skin), nerve damage, and infections are possible risks of breast reduction surgery.

One unpredictable result of this kind of surgery is the possible loss of the ability to breast-feed. For many women, this gamble is enough to dissuade them from getting the surgery.

Rhinoplasty

As with any surgery, there is a risk of infection. What are some of the risks the doctors don't tell you? Take a look at some of the items on a consent form that doctors have patients sign: As with any surgery, death could occur. The sensation in your nose could be permanently altered or it could be lost altogether. There could be breathing obstruction, in which case you will have to undergo another surgical procedure so you can breath again. There could also be nasal septal perforation (a hole in your septum). There is a risk of swelling, bruising, discomfort, infection, and scarring. The swelling may not go down for months after the surgery. Also, there is no guarantee that the results will be symmetrical.

Rhytidectomy

As with any cosmetic surgery, there are risks involved with getting a face-lift. These risks include reactions to anesthesia such as problems breathing, cardiac arrest, and death. Bleeding, infection, hematoma, and injury to the nerves that control facial muscles can also occur.

Chapter 4

What Everyone Should Know About Cosmetic Surgery

Patients have a hard time sorting out who is and is not board certified. "This is confusing for the public," said Dr. Russell Palmer, president of the Plastic Surgery Society's Broward County, Florida, chapter. "Many people want to call themselves 'board-certified' plastic surgeons and so they create their own board. It's troubling."

There is no one organization that exists to monitor the problems with cosmetic surgery. There are several organizations in the United States and Canada that do try to keep current with what the latest trends are in cosmetic surgery.

Who Regulates the Standards of Cosmetic Surgery?

◎ **American Board of Plastic Surgery**

- American Board of Facial Plastic and Reconstructive Surgery

- American Society of Plastic Surgeons (ASPS)

- The American Society for Aesthetic Plastic Surgery

When a Doctor Claims He or She Is Board Certified

An article in *Ladies' Home Journal*, which ran in June 2000, had this cautionary tale about doctors who were "board certified": Leah Carlson, forty-two, did not question the credentials of Dr. Bruce Hildreth, a board-certified emergency-room doctor who became a liposuction specialist. "He had certificates in his office from the American Academy of Cosmetic Surgery and the American Society of Liposuction Surgery (ASLSS)," said Carlson.

The ASLSS is a subgroup of the American Academy of Cosmetic Surgery that sends a certificate to any licensed doctor who pays the membership fee and has taken an approved course in liposuction that lasts at least fourteen hours.

In June 1995, Carlson paid Dr. Hildreth $3,300 to remove fat from her thighs and buttocks. The surgery failed to make a noticeable improvement, so Hildreth offered to do a second procedure four months later, for free. "The results were gruesome," said Carlson. "My knees were painfully swollen, and when I took a bath, skin peeled off my thighs. I ran out of the bathroom screaming," she said.

Dr. Hildreth treated Carlson for a month at his office with antibiotic cream, and he drained fluid from her legs with a syringe. Her condition didn't improve. She developed gigantic seromas, a complication that occurs when fat removal leaves gaps between skin and muscle that fill the body with fluid. Leah Carlson now has twenty-inch-long scars on her legs.

Why Board Certification?

The American Board of Plastic Surgery is a member board of the American Board of Medical Specialties. There are specific and detailed training procedures that plastic surgeons must go through before they can qualify for board certification. That means that, before becoming certified, plastic surgeons must pass written and oral tests to prove that they have understood the training and can perform the procedures of plastic surgery. The American Board of Plastic Surgery is one of twenty-four accredited specialty boards recognized by the American Board of Medical Specialties.

Once a certificate from the American Board of Plastic Surgery is obtained, it must be renewed every ten years. This is to make sure that plastic surgery practitioners keep up-to-date with the newest and safest medical technology.

Cosmetic Surgery and Medical Malpractice: Frequently Asked Questions

What Is Medical Malpractice?

Medical malpractice is behavior by a doctor or other health-care provider that is negligent. A doctor's behavior is considered negligent when he or she fails to follow accepted professional standards of care, and that care, or lack of it, causes harm to the patient.

What Is Informed Consent?

Except in the case of an emergency, a doctor must get a patient's agreement to any course of treatment. Doctors must tell the patient anything that would affect the patient's decision. Informed consent varies from state to state, but generally the doctors explain the nature of the treatment, its risks, side effects, and results, and other courses of action that are reasonable. Some states let older minors give consent to certain procedures.

Who Makes a Living from Cosmetic Surgery?

Doctors

An article in southern Florida's *Sun-Sentinel* cited this figure on the earnings of doctors involved in cosmetic surgery: One in four plastic surgeons nationwide took home $300,000 or more in 1997, according to a survey by *Medical Economics* magazine.

Doctors can make so much money doing cosmetic surgery that one of their sales tactics is to discount their procedures. "One of the staff members gave me a price of $6,500," recalled Jacqueline Lewis in a June 2000 article in *Ladies' Home Journal*. Lewis wanted a breast reduction, but she was nervous about surgery and the cost of the procedure and decided to postpone her final decision. "I told them I needed to think it over. First they sent a letter saying they had a weekend special for $5,000, then they sent a second letter a week later knocking the price down to $4,500."

Lewis went through with the surgery, but suffered for it. She wanted to reduce her 44DD breasts to a size 36C, but after the surgery, "I couldn't fill a 36C bra—my goal—or even a B," she said. Also, Lewis lost her nipples because after the surgeon had removed them, he couldn't put them back. The skin graft failed because the surgeon hadn't had enough experience in doing nipple grafts.

Lawyers

There are some lawyers who specialize in medical malpractice suits, and they have a booming business on hand when it comes to cosmetic surgery. The highly risky nature of cosmetic surgery, added to the fact that it is not regulated in many states the way it needs to be for patient safety, ensures that there will always be medical malpractice lawsuits in this area.

The *Sun-Sentinel* quoted two lawyers who are familiar with medical malpractice suits. "The system is failing consumers," said W. M. Chanfrau, a Daytona Beach, Florida, lawyer who represented eight patients who have sued a local plastic surgeon. "There is no incentive for the medical profession to clean up its act," he said.

"We see everything—tummy tucks gone bad, breasts deformed after implant surgery. It's unbelievable," said a Fort Lauderdale, Florida, attorney who specializes in medical malpractice.

Cosmetic Surgery: Not Just for the Rich Anymore

According to figures published in the 1992 *American Society for Plastic and Reconstructive Surgeons Guide to Cosmetic Surgery*, the most recent statistics available, 30 percent of cosmetic surgery patients had household incomes of less than $25,000 a year. Another

35 percent earned household incomes between $25,000 and $50,000 a year.

How to Finance Cosmetic Surgery

Some plans, like the Colorado-based MediCredit and Tynion's Unicorn Financial Services, are offered to the patient by the doctor after the surgery is set up. The finance companies buy the contracts from the doctors and space the payments out over time at an annual interest rate that can range, depending on the plan and the patient, from about 9 percent to about 20 percent (which is higher than most credit cards).

There are other plans to finance cosmetic surgery. Two are Cooperative Images and Jayhawk. These plans work a little differently from the ones offered in doctors' offices. They sign up a bunch of doctors who are willing to work for a discounted payment. In return, the companies take over the responsibility of getting business for the doctors. Many people have undergone cosmetic surgery procedures for which they literally will be paying the rest of their lives.

Chapter 5

Cosmetic Surgery Horror Stories

The dangers involved in cosmetic surgery are scary—and real. Many people don't think they could become part of the growing percentage of cosmetic surgery patients who have had disastrous things happen as a result of an improperly done procedure. Read on to find out some of the gruesome results of cosmetic surgeries gone wrong.

Penile Enlargement Gone Awry

OnHealth, a Web-based magazine, ran an article in July 1999 about a man in Texas whose complications from a penile lengthening procedure put him in the hospital for ten days, receiving an antibiotic by IV. "If the infection didn't clear up, I faced castration," he said.

Jerry, a fifty-five-year-old from Los Angeles, had a penile enlargement process done. After his first surgery, Jerry developed a serious infection and woke in the middle of the night to see a quarter-inch hole in the side of his penis with "fat cells streaming out."

The Associated Press reported that more than fifty men who went for penile enlargement to Dr. Melvyn Rosenstein, a surgeon in California, have gone to attorneys, complaining about numbness, deformity, and dysfunction. These patients are suing for fraud, medical negligence, and false advertising. Dr. Rosenstein's advertisements claimed false promises about what the surgery could do. Many of these men came down with raging infections because there were sterility problems in the office.

All About Liposuction Gone Horribly Wrong

Edward Mondeck's wife, Rosemarie, thirty-nine, had a bit of tummy fat removed with tumescent liposuction. Rosemarie went into cardiac arrest and died. "It was supposed to be a touch-up procedure," said Mondeck. "All she had was a fatty area above her bellybutton."

On March 17, 1997, a forty-seven-year-old California woman died at Irvine Medical Center after a massive procedure: ten and a half hours of liposuction on her legs, hips, thighs, buttocks, knees, and arms, plus a face-lift. Her plastic surgeon gave her too much tumescent fluid, according to a 2000 article in *U.S. News and World Report*, which resulted in her death.

U.S. News and World Report published an article on February 21, 2000, about Lisa Marie Marinelli of Beachwood, New Jersey. She was a twenty-three-year-old secretary who went to a dermatologist because of a rash. She made an appointment for liposuction after having read a brochure about the procedure in the doctor's waiting room. Doctor Rami Geffner of Toms River, New Jersey, removed a small amount of fat from the young woman's knees and thighs, and then wrapped her legs in Ace bandages. The next day, Lisa was dead from a blood clot in the lung. "My daughter died for two tablespoons of fat," the grieving mother said.

In 1998, the *Toronto Star* published an article that included information about Sandra Ciuffreda, a patient who arranged to have liposuction at the La Fontaine Cosmetic Surgery Center in Canada. The clinic helped her get a $10,000 loan for the surgery, and in October 1997, she had 4.75 gallons of fat sucked from her body. She was sent home hours later, weak and disoriented. "I was in such pain," said Ciuffreda. When she took off the bandages, "There was this huge open wound underneath." Today, she has an inch-wide, ten-inch-long scar.

"Too Much, Too Soon" Cosmetic Surgery

An article in *Cosmopolitan* that ran in 1997 cited the case of Julia, who started changing her face at age eighteen. She has had her nose done twice. She has had tiny scars on her face filled with collagen and silicone, her skin has been refined with dermabrasion, and she has had a silicone chin implant. She has had her lips reinflated three times: first with collagen, then with fat from her own buttocks, and the third time with silicone.

In the same article, it was stated that there are other dangers with "too much, too soon" surgery: It can make a young person look older. Actress Tori Spelling is the current poster girl for this problem. "She was shopping around for her umpteenth nose job," says one doctor, "and I said 'please count me out.' It's impossible to tell what age she is. You wouldn't know if she was a twentysomething trying to look more sophisticated or a thirty-five-year-old trying to look younger. It's spooky, like something out of *The Twilight Zone.*"

The Terrible Quest for Thinner Thighs

An article in *Ladies' Home Journal* in June 2000 cited the case of Ellen Ross, a thirty-seven-year-old woman who wanted thinner thighs. She went to the Center for Cosmetic Surgery in Fort Lauderdale and saw Dr. Leon Doyan, who convinced her to have her buttocks and knees done as well. About two weeks later, after she had been sedated in preparation for surgery, Dr. Doyan convinced Ross to have another procedure for an extra $500.

"He looked at my breasts and said they were a six but he could make them a ten by injecting the fat he was removing into my cleavage," said Ross. Ross agreed. The results were horrifying. "I had lumps next to my breasts," she said. Dr. Doyan said that he couldn't extract enough fat during the procedure to finish augmenting her breasts, and he suggested fixing the problem with a $1,500 implant operation, which she did undergo. She developed such a serious infection after the implant surgery that she needed a double mastectomy and eighteen reconstructive operations. Her breasts are scarred to this day. She sued and was awarded $1.8 million, but she never collected a cent because Dr. Doyan claimed bankruptcy and had no medical malpractice insurance.

A Flesh-Eating Bug

Cosmetic surgery can be very dangerous, as one patient knows only too well. She does not want to reveal her identity, but last year she went in for abdominoplasty, better known as a tummy tuck. Soon after surgery, she contracted necrotising fasicitis, a potentially fatal infection caused by a flesh-eating bug. If it can't be treated with antibiotics, the infected area has to be surgically removed, which results in substantial scarring. After her original operation, she had to have eleven operations.

The New York State Senate Committee on the Risks of Office Surgery

In February 1999, the New York State Senate Committee conducted an investigation of cosmetic surgery performed in offices rather than in hospitals. What the committee found was shocking.

◎ **Compared to a hospital or an ambulatory surgical center, an office is the most dangerous place in which to undergo anesthesia.**

◎ **Anesthesia equipment in offices is frequently out-of-date or poorly kept. In fact, some physicians purchase old anesthesia machines for their offices, which have been discarded by hospitals because they are not up to code.**

◎ **In New York, any person with a medical license can advertise that he or she does liposuction or performs other cosmetic procedures. Some doctors may perform such procedures with no more preparation than a three-day weekend seminar or a thirty-minute videotaped training session.**

⊙ Marathon operations for multiple
   procedures, which include many hours
   of general anesthesia, invite cardiovas-
   cular distress.

Cosmetic Surgery: Risky Business

So, do you still think that having cosmetic surgery is a glamorous thing? This book has clearly shown that, although people want to get cosmetic surgery to become more attractive, many times cosmetic surgery can leave you damaged, disfigured, or dead. There is nothing attractive in those options!

The data that has been collected about the dangers of cosmetic surgery is frightening enough. It is more frightening still to realize that these horrible statistics may be just a small part of the cosmetic surgery disasters that actually do occur more often than are reported. Even the FDA does not have enough data to rule cosmetic surgery safe and effective across the board. If you find yourself considering cosmetic surgery as an option, consider that what we know about its risks is awful, and that the reality of it could be much, much worse.

Glossary

abscess Swollen, inflamed area of the body in which pus gathers.

anesthesia Medicine used to produce numbness, loss of feeling, or unconsciousness.

blepharoplasty Surgical reshaping of the eyelid.

blood clot A lump formed when blood coagulates, or sticks together.

body dysmorphic disorder Disorder in which people obsess about small flaws in their bodies.

cardiac arrest When the heart stops beating.

cardiac arrhythmia Abnormal heartbeat caused by heart disease and high blood pressure.

cartilage Tough tissue in the body of which structures like the ears and the nose are partially made.

dermabrasion Technique for removing the upper layers of skin.

epinephrine Hormone secreted by the adrenal gland that increases heart rate and muscular strength.

face-lift Surgery performed to remove sagging skin and wrinkles from a patient's face.

hematoma When blood collects at a surgical site.

lidocaine Type of anesthesia.

liposuction Surgical technique for removing fat from under the skin by vacuum suctioning.

peritonitis Inflammation of the peritoneum, the smooth membrane that lines the cavity of the abdomen.

pulmonary thromboemboli Common complication caused when blood clots lodge in the lungs.

reconstructive surgery Correction of an abnormality caused by birth defects, disease, or traumatic injury.

rhinoplasty Surgery done to change the shape of the nose.

tissue Bunches of cells. Tissues make up organs of the body.

ultrasound wand Tool that uses ultrasonic waves (waves of a frequency so high that humans can't hear them), sometimes for the purposes of surgery.

Where to Go for Help

In the United States

American Academy of Dermatology
930 N. Meacham Road
P.O. Box 4014
Schaumburg, IL 60168-4014
(847) 330-0230
Web site: http://www.aad.org

American Academy of Facial Plastic and
    Reconstructive Surgery
310 S. Henry Street
Alexandria, VA 22314
(800) 332-3223
Web site: http://www.facial-plastic-surgery.org

American Board of Plastic Surgery
Seven Penn Center, Suite 400
1635 Market Street
Philadelphia, PA 19103-2204
(215) 587-9322
e-mail: info@abplsurg.org
Web site: http://www.abplsurg.org

In Canada

Canadian Academy of Facial Plastic
 and Reconstructive Surgery
Mount Sinai Hospital
600 University Avenue, Room 401
Toronto, ON M5G 1X5
(800) 545-8864
e-mail: info@facialcosmeticsurgery.org
Web site: http://www.facialcosmeticsurgery.org

Canadian Medical Association
1867 Alta Vista Drive
Ottawa, ON K1G 3Y6
(613) 731-9331
e-mail: public_affairs@cma.ca
Web site: http://www.cma.ca

Canadian Society for Aesthetic (Cosmetic)
 Plastic Surgery
2334 Heska Road

Pickering, ON L1V 2P9
(905) 831-7750
e-mail: information@csaps.ca
Web site: http://www.csaps.ca

Web Sites
The American Society for Aesthetic Plastic Surgery
http://www.surgery.org

The International Plastic, Reconstructive,
    and Aesthetic Foundation
http://worldplasticsurgery.org/ipraf/index.html

Plastic Surgery Information Service
http://www.plasticsurgery.org

For Further Reading

Angell, Marcia. *Science on Trial: The Clash of Medical Evidence and the Law in the Breast Implant Case.* New York: W.W. Norton & Company, 1997.

Davis, Kathy. *Reshaping the Female Body: The Dilemma of Cosmetic Surgery.* New York: Routledge Books, 1995.

Gail, Susan. *Cosmetic Surgery: Before, Between, and After.* Holt, MI: Partners Publishers Group, Inc., 2000.

Ganny, Charlee, and Susan J. Collini. *Two Girlfriends Get Real About Cosmetic Surgery.* Los Angeles: Renaissance Books, 2000.

Loftus, Jean M. *The Smart Woman's Guide to Plastic Surgery: Essential Information from a Female Plastic Surgeon.* Lincolnwood, IL: Contemporary Books, 2000.

Marfuggi, Richard A. *Plastic Surgery: What You Need to Know Before, During, and After.* New York: Perigee Books, 1998.

Nash, Joyce D. *What Your Doctor Can't Tell You About Cosmetic Surgery.* Lincoln, NE: iUniverse.com, Inc., 2000.

Stewart, Mary White. *Silicone Spills: Breast Implants on Trial.* Westport, CT: Praeger Publishers Trade, 1998.

Sullivan, Deborah A. *Cosmetic Surgery: The Cutting Edge of Commercial Medicine in America.* New Brunswick, NJ: Rutgers University Press, 2001.

Index

About the Author
Magdalena Alagna is an editor and freelance writer living in New York City.

Photo Credits
Cover, pp. 2, 17, 37 © Corbis; pp. 10, 23, 29, 32 © Custom Medical Stock Photo; p. 14 © Associated Press.

Book Designer
Nelson Sa